Keto Alcohol Drinks

Easy Keto Cocktails Recipes for Beginners you Can Enjoy at Home with Your Friends to Lose Weight and Burn Fat

Jenny Kern

Table Of Contents

Introduction

Thank you for purchasing this book. So, you've had a long, tiring day at the office and are mentally and physically drained. The only thing on your mind right now is to crawl into your favorite bar, say hello to your usual bartender, and order a nice and tasty cocktail to help you kick back and unwind. For years, cocktails, those delicious alcoholic blends, have been helping tense and stressed people relax and unwind. However, how many of these drinkers know how to make them themselves? In this book we will follow you step by step to create your favorite cocktails. I hope you like them.

Enjoy.

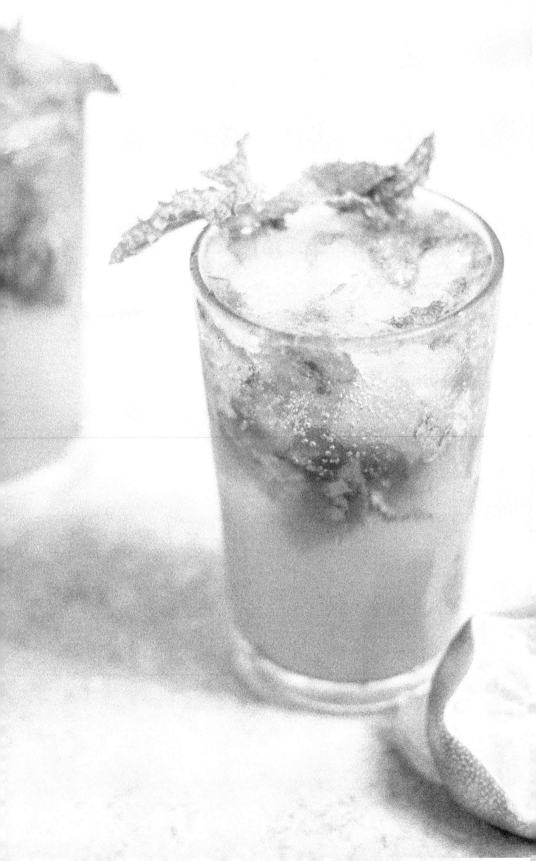

Wine and Champagne Keto Cocktails

Lava Champagne with Gelatin

Preparation time: 10 minutes

Servings: 6

Ingredients:

1 750-ml. bottle champagne

1 c. vodka

1 c. boiling water

1 3-oz. package blue or red instant Jell-O mix

Directions:

Mix the boiling water and gelatin mix in a bowl for around two minutes or until the mixture completely dissolves.

Pour in the vodka. Pour this liquid mixture into individual portions or small paper cups. Chill in the fridge for approximately two hours or until set.

Once the gelatin mixture is set, pour the champagne into cocktail glasses. Use a fork to break up the gelatin.

Add the mixture to a glass of champagne. Stir it gradually to produce some lava action. Serve and enjoy.

Raspberry cocktail

Preparation time: 10 minutes

Servings: 4

Ingredients:

2 bottles of cold sparkling wine of excellent quality, if you like you can choose it more or less sweet

4 spoons of sugar

4 little boxes of fresh raspberries, or an equivalent quantity of frozen raspberries

Directions:

Pour the wine, which, as mentioned, must be very cold, into a decorative container, for example, a crystal or silver bowl. Pour in the sugar, and give it a stir. Add the raspberries.

Serve as an aperitif, using a silver ladle to pour in cups or flutes.

Bishop Cocktail

Preparation time: 10 minutes

Servings: 3

Ingredients:

30 milliliters orange juice

2 teaspoons runny honey

75 milliliters tawny port wine

90 milliliters boiling water

7 cloves

Directions:

Use preheated heat-proof glass. Muddle cloves in the base of the shaker. Put in boiling water and stir in honey and other ingredients. Strain into glass. Use grated nutmeg to garnish.

Orange punch

Preparation time: 30 minutes

Servings: 4

Ingredients:

4 cups of water

25oz. of sugar

3 cups of Aperol

3 untreated oranges

Directions:

To prepare the punch, wash and dry the oranges well, peel them with the help of a peeler, then keep the peel aside.

Cut fruit in half and squeeze them using a juicer, then strain the juice and put it in a large bowl.

Prepare the syrup now: in a saucepan, heat the sugar with the water, and cook everything over low heat until the sugar has completely dissolved. Meanwhile, add Aperol to the orange juice.

When ready, add the sugar syrup. Finally, add the orange peel (which you had previously kept aside) and leave to infuse for a few minutes. Serve the punch still hot.

Tips:

Store the punch in the refrigerator, closed in an airtight container, for a maximum of 3-4 days. When serving, heat it in a saucepan.

Frozen peach champagne cocktail

Preparation time: 10 minutes

Servings: 4

Ingredients:

4ml of Alize peach

1 cup ice

12ml chilled champagne

3 tablespoons powdered sugar

2 cups frozen peach slices

2 tablespoons grenadine

Directions:

Mix frozen peaches, powdered sugar, Alize peach, and ice in a blender. Blend the mixture and add champagne until it smoothens

Pour in the remaining champagne and stir it thoroughly

Place in each glass ¼ of the mixture then take a tablespoon of grenadine and add to each of the glasses. On top add the remaining peach mixture

Garnish then serve.

Basil and Pomegranate Champagne Cocktail

Preparation time: 10 minutes

Servings: 4

Ingredients:

2 fresh basil leaves

4-fl. oz. champagne

1 tbsp. pomegranate juice

Directions:

Put the basil leaves in the bottom of the champagne flute. Add the pomegranate juice.

Muddle the leaves lightly to release their flavor. Top the mixture with champagne. Serve.

Peach Blossom Champagne

Preparation time: 10 minutes

Servings: 8

Ingredients:

2/3 c. peach schnapps

5 c. orange juice

2 c. ice cubes

1 tbsp. grenadine syrup

1 ½ c. champagne, chilled

Optional ingredient: 6 peach slices

Directions:

Mix peach schnapps and orange juice in a pitcher. Place in your fridge for around thirty minutes or until chilled.

Pour a half-cup of the mixture into 6 glasses. Add around two to three ice cubes into each glass.

Add three to four tablespoons of champagne per glass. Drizzle a half teaspoon of the grenadine syrup into each glass. Do not stir. If you are using peach slices, garnish each drink with one slice. Serve.

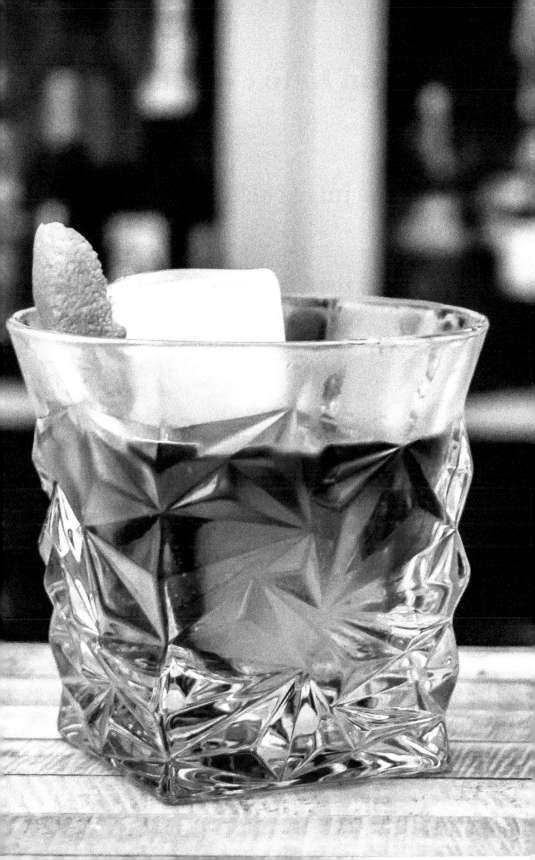

Gin Keto Cocktails

Orange juice cocktail

Preparation time: 10 minutes

Servings: 6

Ingredients:

4 cups of Prosecco or Spumante Brut

1/2 cup of gin

1/2 cup of natural orange juice from fresh oranges

2 teaspoons of sugar (optional)

Directions:

Squeeze the oranges.

Divide the juice into cold cocktail glasses (preferably flute or hurricane), passing it directly through a colander.

Then add the Spumante Brut or Prosecco.

Also, add the gin in the 6 glasses, if you want - add the sugar, mix, and serve.

Tips:

You can decorate the glass with orange slices and dip a cherry in alcohol.

Champagne pink cocktail

Preparation time: 15 minutes

Servings: 2

Calories: 109 Kcal

Ingredients:

2 pieces of candied ginger

0.5oz. of sugar

2 tablespoons of fruit and ginger syrup

1 cup of very cold rosé champagne

6oz. of mixed candied fruit

2 cups of water

5 tablespoons of orange vodka

ice cubes to taste

Directions:

Prepare the fruit and ginger syrup in advance.

Bring the water to a boil, then throw in the candied fruit, ginger, and sugar.

Simmer gently for 5 minutes, then let cool.

Blend everything with a powerful mixer until a homogeneous mixture is obtained.

Pass through a sieve and refrigerate in an air-tight container until ready to use.

To prepare the cocktail, pour the vodka, the mixture obtained, and two tablespoons of syrup into a shaker filled with ice. Shake with energy.

Fill two flutes with champagne and then complete them with the contents of the shaker passed through the strainer. Serve immediately.

Devil Twister

Preparation time: 10 minutes

Servings: 2

Ingredients:

8 milliliters Fernet Branca

8 milliliters triple sec

15 milliliters cold water

15 milliliters Dubonnet Red

60 milliliters London dry gin

Directions:

Shake ingredients with ice and strain into chilled glass. Garnish using lemon zest twist.

Destiny

Preparation time: 10 minutes

Servings: 2

Ingredients:

8 milliliters lemon juice

8 milliliters sugar syrup

15 milliliters crème de cassis

15 milliliters vanilla liqueur

30 milliliters London dry gin

90 milliliters cranberry juice

6 fresh blackberries

Directions:

Muddle blackberries in the base of the shaker. Put in other ingredients, shake with ice, and strain into a glass filled with crushed ice. Garnish using mint.

Crash Impact

Preparation time: 10 minutes

Servings: 2

Ingredients:

8 milliliters triple sec

15 milliliters dry vermouth

15 milliliters sweet vermouth8 milliliters lemon juice

2 dashes bitters

60 milliliters London dry gin

Directions:

Shake ingredients with ice and strain into chilled glass. Garnish using maraschino cherry.

Country Breeze

Preparation time: 10 minutes

Servings: 2

Ingredients:

15 milliliters crème de cassis

60 milliliters London dry gin

105 milliliters apple juice

Directions:

Shake ingredients with ice and strain into ice-filled glass. Garnish using strawberries and blueberries.

Alexander Cocktail

Preparation time: 10 minutes

Servings: 2

Ingredients:

15 milliliters whipping cream

30 milliliters white crème de cacao liqueur

60 milliliters London dry gin

Directions:

Shake ingredients with ice and strain into chilled glass. Garnish using grated nutmeg.

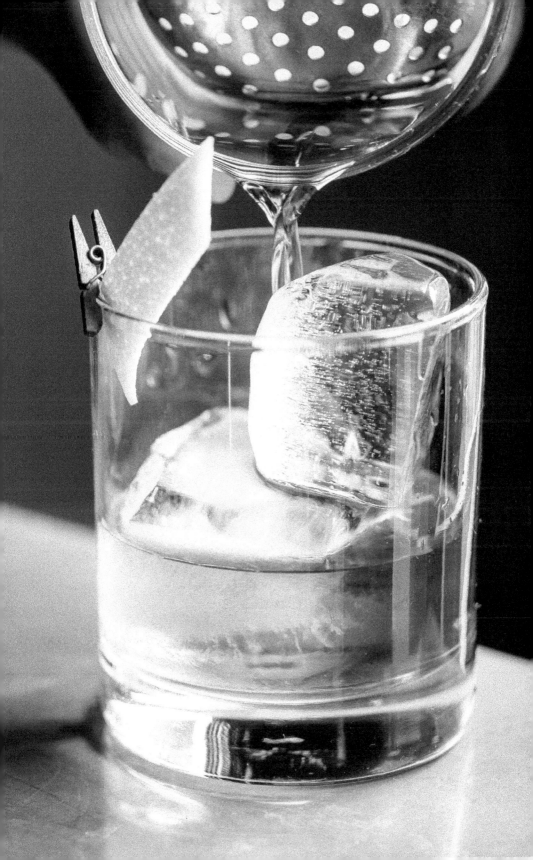

Whiskey Keto Cocktails

Original Irish Cream

Preparation time: 15 minutes

Servings: 12

Ingredients:

1 cup heavy cream

1 (14 oz.) can sweetened condensed milk

1 2/3 cups Irish whiskey

1 tsp. instant coffee granules

2 tbsps. chocolate syrup

1 tsp. vanilla extract

1 tsp. almond extract

Directions:

Mix almond extract, vanilla extract, chocolate syrup, instant coffee, Irish whiskey, sweetened condensed milk, and heavy cream in a blender.

Blend for 20-30 seconds on the high setting.

Keep in a tightly sealed container in the fridge. Shake thoroughly before serving.

St. Michael's Irish Americano

Preparation time: 10 minutes

Servings: 2

Ingredients:

2 (1.5 fluid oz.) jiggers espresso coffee

2 (1.5 fluid oz.) jiggers Irish whiskey

1 tbsp. white sugar

1 tbsp. heavy cream

6 fluid oz. hot water

2 tbsps. whipped cream, garnish

Directions:

In your favorite mug, pour the espresso in then put in hot water, tbsp. cream, sugar, and Irish whiskey.

Use a dollop of whipped cream to garnish.

Shamrock

Preparation time: 10 minutes

Servings: 2

Ingredients:

15 milliliters cold water

15 milliliters green Chartreuse

15 milliliters green crème de menthe

45 milliliters dry vermouth

45 milliliters Irish whiskey

Directions:

Shake ingredients with ice and strain into chilled glass. Garnish using mint.

Rat Pack Manhattan

Preparation time: 10 minutes

Servings: 2

Ingredients:

15 milliliters Grand Marnier

22 milliliters dry vermouth

22 milliliters sweet vermouth

45 milliliters bourbon whiskey

3 dashes bitters

Directions:

Chill glass, add Grand Marnier, swirl to coat and then discard. Stir other ingredients with ice and strain into liqueur-coated glass. Garnish using orange zest twist and maraschino cherry.

Quebec

Preparation time: 10 minutes

Servings: 2

Ingredients:

2 dashes of orange bitters

60 milliliters Canadian whiskey

60 milliliters Dubonnet Red

Directions:

Stir ingredients and strain into chilled glass. Garnish using orange zest twist.

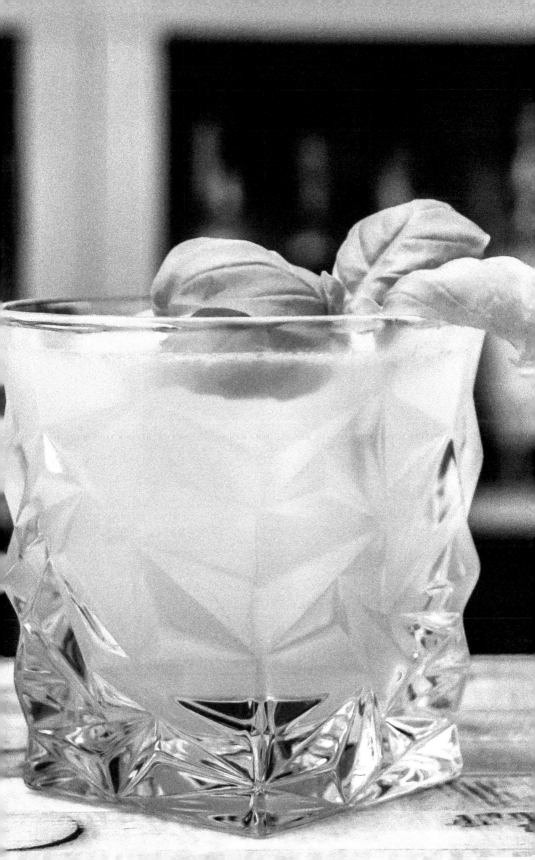

Tequila Cocktails

Sangrita

Preparation time: 10 minutes

Servings: 5

Ingredients:

¼ cup fresh lime juice

1 cup orange juice

2 cups tomato juice

2 teaspoons chopped onion

2 teaspoons hot sauce

2 teaspoons Worcestershire sauce

lime wedges, for serving

salt and freshly ground black pepper to taste

shot of pure agave tequila (a silver tequila is preferable because its agave bite complements the spicy sangrita)

Directions:

Mix the lime juice, onion, hot sauce, Worcestershire, and salt and pepper in a blender.

Blend until the desired smoothness is achieved.

In a pitcher, mix the mixed mixture with the orange juice and tomato juice.

Chill.

Before you serve, stir thoroughly, pour into little glasses, and pour tequila into separate shot glasses.

Drink the tequila, suck on a lime wedge, and chase it with the sangrita.

Mango Sangrita

Preparation time: 10 minutes

Servings: 2

Ingredients:

1 ounce Fresh Sour

1 ounce mango puree

1 teaspoon Tabasco

1½ ounces silver tequila

2 ounces tomato juice

Directions:

Mix all of the ingredients in a cocktail shaker with ice and stir contents.

Strain into a shot glass or martini glass.

Reverse Wind

Preparation time: 10 minutes

Servings: 2

Ingredients:

½ fresh egg white

15 milliliters maple syrup

22 milliliters lemon juice

2 dashes bitters

60 milliliters tequila

Directions:

Shake ingredients with ice and strain into chilled glass. Garnish using lemon zest twist.

Requiem Daiquiri

Preparation time: 10 minutes

Servings: 2

Ingredients:

8 milliliters navy rum

8 milliliters sugar syrup

15 milliliters lime juice

30 milliliters tequila

Directions:

Shake ingredients with ice and strain into chilled glass. Garnish using a lime wedge.

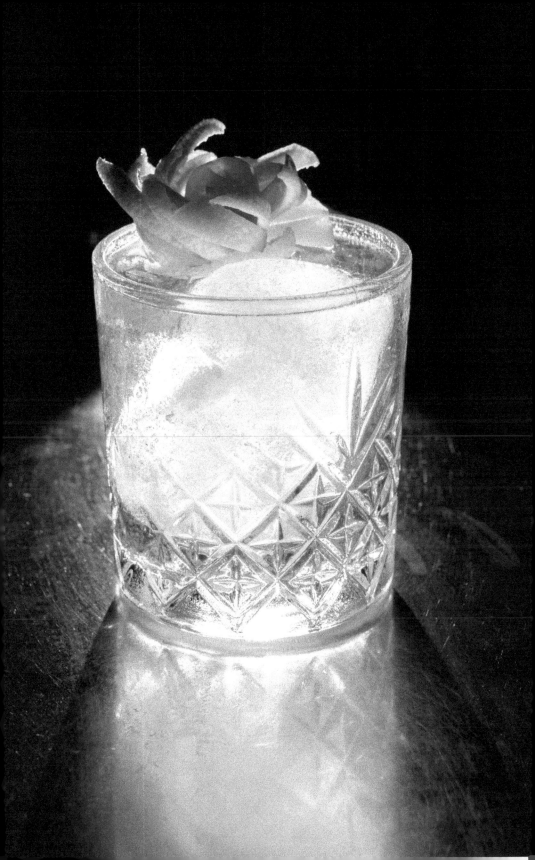

Rum Keto Cocktails

Piña colada

Preparation time: 10 minutes

Servings: 2

Ingredients:

60 ml (2 oz.) white rum

120 ml (4 oz.) pineapple juice

60 ml (2 oz.) coconut cream

Pineapple wedges, to garnish

Directions:

Process all the ingredients along with some ice in a blender, until you get a smooth texture.

Pour into a tall glass.

Garnish with some pineapple wedges.

Frozen Strawberry Daiquiri

Preparation time: 10 minutes

Servings: 6

Ingredients:

100 ml (3.4 oz.) rum

200 g (6.8 oz.) ice

500 g (17 oz.) strawberries

The juice of ½ lime

Lime slices, to garnish

1 strawberry, halved, to garnish

Directions:

Blend the strawberries until you get a creamy texture, and remove all seeds.

Put the puree into the blender with rum, lime juice, and ice.

Divide the blended mixture between 2 Martini glasses.

Garnish with lime slices and strawberry halves.

Apple Cooler

Preparation time: 5 minutes

Servings: 2

Ingredients:

2 oz. white rum

4 oz. apple juice

2 oz. Sprite

Ice

Apple, for garnish

Directions:

Fill a highball glass to the top with ice

Pour in 3 ½ oz. of apple juice and 1 ½ oz. of white rum

Top up with Sprite and stir gently

Garnish with 3 apple wedges

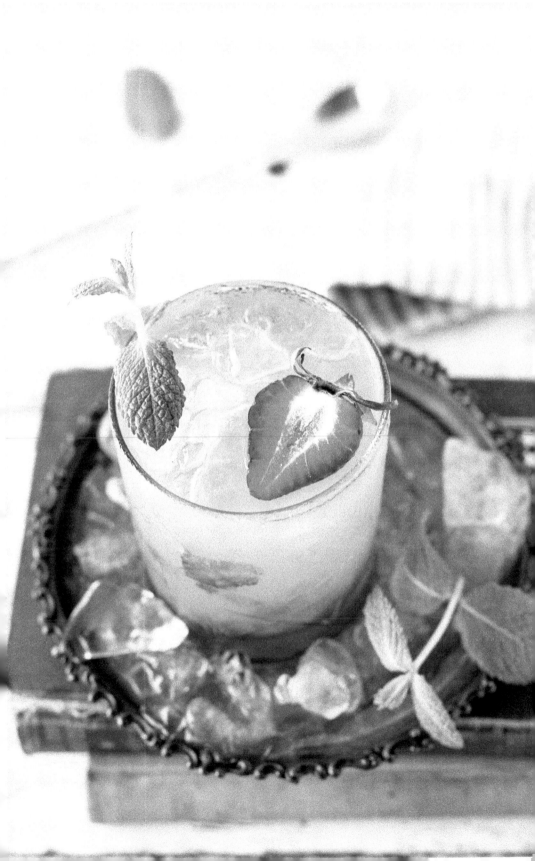

Vodka Keto Cocktails

Frozen special Martini

Preparation time: 10 minutes

Servings: 2

Ingredients:

1 oz. vodka

1 oz. coffee liqueur

1½ oz. espresso coffee

¼ oz. vanilla syrup

Ice

Coffee beans, for garnish

Directions:

Pour 1½ oz. of chilled espresso, ¼ oz. of vanilla syrup, 1 oz. of coffee liqueur, and 1 oz. of vodka into a shaker

Fill the shaker with ice cubes and shake

Garnish with coffee beans after straining in a chilled glass

Moscow Mule

Preparation time: 5 minutes

Servings: 2

Ingredients:

2 oz. of vodka, classic

3 oz. of beer, ginger

1/2 lime, juice only, fresh

For garnishing – 1 lime wedge, fresh

Directions:

Add the vodka, then ginger beer & lime juice to a copper cocktail mug or a highball glass.

Fill the mug or glass using crushed ice.

Stir to combine well.

Use lime wedge for garnishing and serve.

Dirty Martini

Preparation time: 10 minutes

Servings: 2

Ingredients:

6 ounces vodka

1 ounce olive brine

1 dash dry vermouth

Ice cubes

4 stuffed green olives

Directions:

Shake vodka, olive brine, and dry vermouth.

Pour into a Collins glass.

Fill with ice cubes.

Garnish with green olives.

Caramel Spiced Tea

Preparation time: 5 minutes

Servings: 2

Ingredients:

1.5 ounces Smirnoff Kissed Caramel vodka

2 ounces unsweetened strong Chai tea

1 ounce half-and-half

0.5 ounces simple syrup

Ice cubes

Directions:

Shake vodka, strong Chai tea, half-and-half, and maple syrup.

Pour into a Collins glass.

Fill with ice cubes.

Pomegranate Berry Punch

Preparation time: 5 minutes

Servings: 2

Ingredients:

1.5 ounces Smirnoff sorbet light raspberry pomegranate vodka

1 ounce cranberry juice

2 ounces cocktail ginger ale

Ice cubes

1 lime wedge

Directions:

Shake Smirnoff vodka, cranberry juice, and cocktail ginger ale

Pour into a Collins glass.

Fill with ice cubes.

Garnish with lime wedges.

Honey Cider

Preparation time: 5 minutes

Servings: 2

Ingredients:

1.5 ounces Smirnoff wild honey vodka

2.5 ounces cider

2.5 ounces apple juice

Ice cubes

Directions:

Shake Smirnoff wild honey, cider, and apple juice.

Pour into a Collins glass.

Fill with ice cubes.

Black Cherry Bloom

Preparation time: 5 minutes

Servings: 2

Ingredients:

1 ounce blood orange Juice

¾ ounce lime juice

¾ ounce agave nectar

2 ounces black cherry vodka

3 sliced strawberry

4 mint leaves

1 pinch cayenne pepper

Ice cubed

For garnishing:

2 mint leaves

1 hulled strawberry

Directions:

Shake cherry vodka, blood orange juice, lime juice, and agave nectar.

Add vodka, strawberry, mint leaves, and cayenne pepper and shake with ice cubes.

Strain into a Collins glass and garnish with mint leaves and strawberry.

Red Tart

Preparation time: 5 minutes

Servings: 2

Ingredients:

1½ ounces red berry vodka

¾ ounce black raspberry liqueur

1 ounce amaretto

½ ounce lime juice

1 ounce lemon-lime soda

Ice cubes

Directions:

Shake vodka, black raspberry liqueur, amaretto, lime juice, and lemon-lime soda.

Pour into a Collins glass.

Fill with ice cubes.

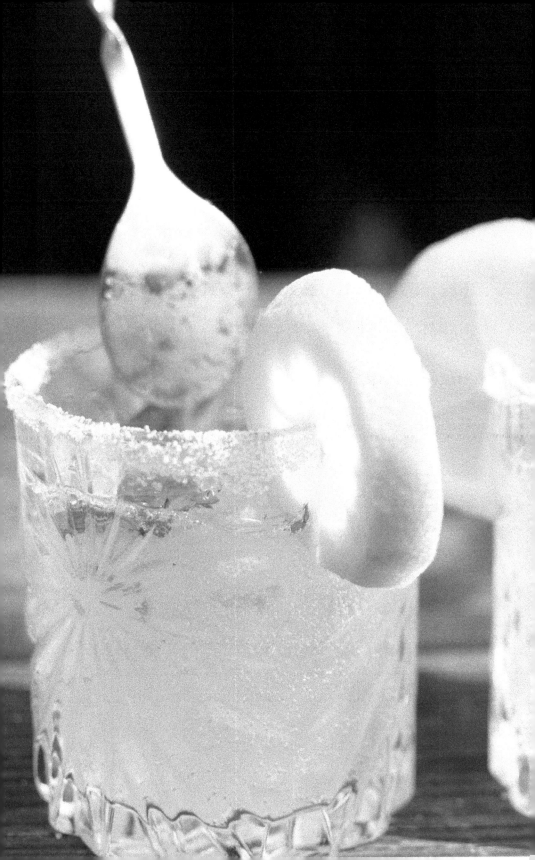

Keto Liqueurs

Benedictine Blast Cocktail

Preparation time: 10 minutes

Servings: 3

Ingredients:

8 milliliters Benedictine D.O.M. liqueur

8 milliliters white crème de cacao liqueur

½ teaspoon mezcal

22 milliliters cold water

60 milliliters tequila

Directions:

Stir ingredients with ice and strain into chilled glass.

Cold Shower

Preparation time: 10 minutes

Servings: 2

Ingredients:

Creme de menthe (1 part, green)

Club soda (4 parts)

Directions:

1. In a highball glass add ice, club soda, and the creme de menthe then stir and enjoy.

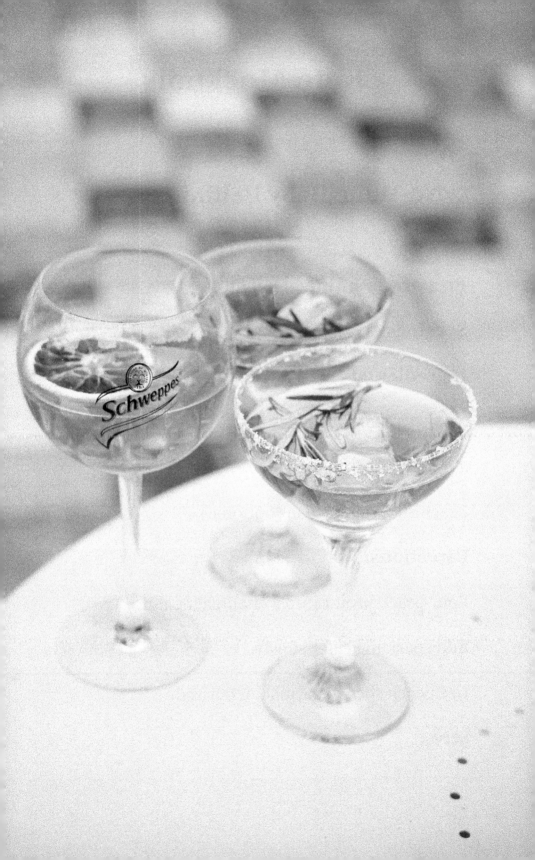

Keto Mocktails

No-Wine Baby Bellini

Preparation time: 4 minutes

Servings: 4

Ingredients:

2 ounces sparkling cider

2 ounces peach nectar

Peach slice for garnish (optional)

Directions:

Pour peach nectar into a champagne flute.

Add sparkling cider slowly.

Use peach slice to garnish, if desired.

Serve.

Orange Basil Mocktail

Preparation time: 10 minutes

Servings: 6

Ingredients:

2 cups orange juice

¼ cup freshly squeezed lemon juice

½ cup soda water

¼ cup water

2 tablespoons sugar

2-3 basil leaves

Ice cubes for serving

Orange slices for garnish

Directions:

In a pitcher, mix orange juice, lemon juice, soda water, water, sugar, and basil.

Spoon ice cubes into serving glasses and pour orange juice on top.

Garnish with orange slices and serve immediately.

Roy Rogers

Preparation time: 10 minutes

Servings: 4

Ingredients:

¼ ounce grenadine

8 ounces cola-flavored soda

1 maraschino strawberry for garnish

Directions:

Fill a tall glass with ice. Pour in grenadine.

Add cola and stir to combine.

Use maraschino strawberry for garnish and serve.

Sherbet Raspberry Mocktail

Preparation time: 10 minutes

Servings: 4

Ingredients:

2 cups Sprite

2 cups soda water

1 (12-ounce) can pink lemonade

½ cup pineapple wedges

½ cup raspberries

8 scoops of raspberry sherbet ice cream, frozen

Directions:

In a large glass bowl, mix the Sprite, soda water, lemonade, pineapple wedges, and raspberries.

Pour the drink into serving glasses and scoop one dollop of the ice cream onto each glass.

Enjoy immediately!

Strawberry Faux Daiquiri

Preparation time: 10 minutes

Servings: 4

Ingredients:

2 large strawberries

1 ½ pints orangeade

Crushed ice

1 small strawberry for garnish

Directions:

Hull strawberries.

Combine the crushed ice, strawberries, and orangeade in a blender.

Blend ingredients well. Pour in a glass.

Use strawberry for garnish.

Serve.

Tropical Fruits

Preparation time: 10 minutes

Servings: 4

Ingredients:

1 ¼ cup chopped strawberries

2 cups sparkling water

2 oranges juiced

Directions:

In a pitcher, add the strawberries and use a muddler to mash the fruits.

Pour in the sparkling water, orange juice, and cover the pitcher with plastic wrap.

Chill in the refrigerator for 2 hours.

Serve the drink in glasses.

Tuscan Fresco

Preparation time: 10 minutes

Servings: 1

Ingredients:

Ice made with filtered water

2 sprigs rosemary

1 ounce peach nectar

1 ounce white cranberry juice

½ ounce fresh orange juice

½ ounce store-bought simple syrup

1 ounce chilled club soda

Directions:

Add ice to the cocktail shaker till full.

Add a sprig of rosemary, along with the simple syrup, orange juice, cranberry juice, and peach nectar.

Shake to thoroughly combine. Strain into ice-filled glass.

Stir club soda. Use the remaining sprig of rosemary to garnish. Serve.

Mandarin Mojito Mocktail

Preparation time: 5 minutes

Servings: 3

Ingredients:

8 fluid oz of Sprite or 7UP

½ of a fluid oz of Mandarin Syrup

½ of a fluid oz of Mojito Mix

5 Mandarin orange segments

3-5 large mint leaves

1 lime

Mandarin orange segments as garnish

Directions:

Cut the lime into at least two wedges.

Place the 2 lime wedges, mint leaves & orange segments into your glass.

Muddle the ingredients.

Now place the rest of the ingredients into the glass.

Stir the drink mixture.

Add the desired amount of ice.

Use additional orange segments for garnish.

Virgin Bloody Mary with Shrimp

Preparation time: 5 minutes

Servings: 3

Ingredients:

22 oz of reduced-sodium V8

1 tsp of horseradish

1 tsp of Worcestershire sauce

1 Tbsp of lemon juice

10 dashes Tabasco

Freshly ground pepper, to taste

Ice cubes

4 cooked shrimp

Directions:

Combine the V8, Worcestershire sauce, horseradish, Tabasco, lemon juice & pepper into a glass jar.

Use the lid and shake.

Place ice into two tall glasses.

Evenly divide the drink mixture between the two glasses.

Use the two shrimp as garnish.

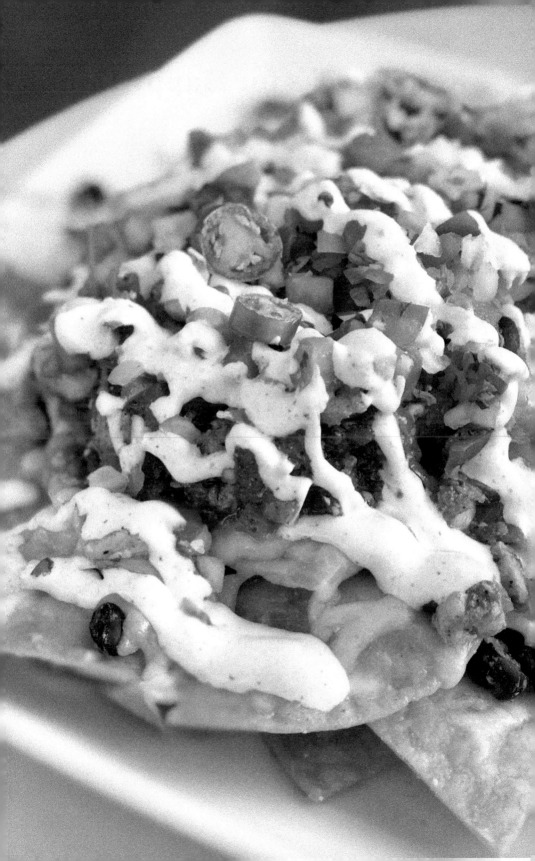

Keto Snacks for Happy Hour

Nutmeg Nougat

Preparation time: 30 minutes

Cooking Time: 60 minutes

Servings: 12

Ingredients:

1 Cup Heavy Cream

1 Cup Cashew Butter

1 Cup Coconut, Shredded

½ Teaspoon Nutmeg

1 Teaspoon Vanilla Extract, Pure

Stevia to Taste

Directions:

Melt your cashew butter using a double boiler, and then stir in your vanilla extract, dairy cream, nutmeg, and stevia. Make sure it's mixed well.

Remove from heat, allowing it to cool down before refrigerating it for half an hour.

Shape into balls, and coat with shredded coconut. Chill for at least two hours before serving.

Nutrition: calories 110, fat 10, fiber 1, carbs 3, protein 6

Sweet Almond Bites

Preparation time: 30 minutes

Cooking Time: 90 minutes

Servings: 12

Ingredients:

18 Ounces Butter, Grass-Fed

2 Ounces Heavy Cream

½ Cup Stevia

2/3 Cup Cocoa Powder

1 Teaspoon Vanilla Extract, Pure

4 Tablespoons Almond Butter

Directions:

Use a double boiler to melt your butter before adding in all of your remaining ingredients.

Place the mixture into molds, freezing for two hours before serving.

Lemon Fat Bombs

Preparation time: 10 minutes

Cooking Time: 50 minutes

Servings: 4

Ingredients:

1 cup of shredded coconut (dry)

1/4 cup of coconut oil

3 tbsps. of erythritol sweetener (powdered)

1 tbsps. of lemon zest

1 pinch of salt

Directions:

Add the coconut to a high-power blender. Blend until creamy for fifteen minutes. Add sweetener, coconut oil, salt, and lemon zest. Blend for two minutes. Fill small muffin cups with the coconut mixture. Chill in the refrigerator for thirty minutes.

Nutrition: calories 200, fat 8, fiber 4, carbs 8, protein 3

Thousand Island Salad Dressing

Preparation time: 5 minutes

Cooking Time: 5 minutes

Servings: 8 servings

Ingredients:

2 Tbsp. olive oil

¼ c frozen spinach, thawed.

2 T dried parsley

1 T dried dill

1 t onion powder

½ t salt

¼ t black pepper

1 c full-fat mayonnaise

¼ c full-fat sour cream

Directions:

Combine all ingredients in a small mixing bowl.

Nutrition: calories 383, fat 14, fiber 4, carbs 3, protein 8

Keto Salad Niçoise

Preparation time: 5 minutes

Cooking Time: 5 minutes

Servings: 4

Ingredients:

2 eggs

2 oz. celery root

4 oz. green beans

2 tablespoons olive oil

2 garlic cloves

4 oz. romaine lettuce

2 oz. cherry tomatoes

¼ red onion

1 can tuna

2 oz. olives

Dressing

2 tablespoons capers

¼ oz. anchovies

½ cup olive oil

½ cup mayonnaise

¼ lemon

1 tablespoon parsley

Directions:

In a bowl sauté peppers in coconut oil. In a bowl add all ingredients and mix well. Serve with dressing

Nutrition: calories 110, fat 10, fiber 1, carbs 3, protein 6

Greek Salad

Preparation time: 5 minutes

Cooking Time: 5 minutes

Servings: 4

Ingredients:

2 ripe tomatoes

¼ cucumber

¼ red onion

¼ green bell pepper

6 oz. feta cheese

8 black Greek olives

5 tablespoons olive oil

¼ tablespoon red wine vinegar

2 tsp oregano

Directions:

In a bowl add all ingredients and mix well. Serve with dressing

Nutrition: calories 383, fat 14, fiber 4, carbs 3, protein 8

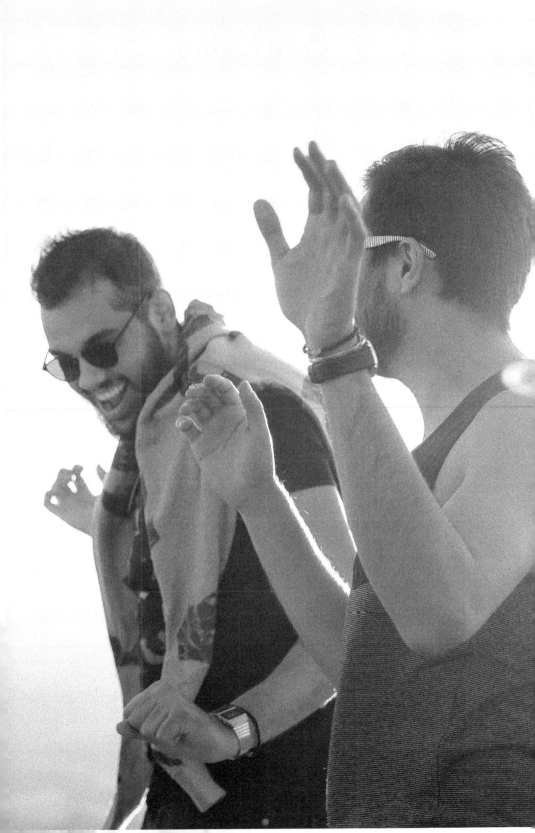

Conclusion

Here we come to the end of our journey with keto cocktails. In addition to being really delicious, these cocktails will also help you lose weight and counteract some diseases. Obviously remember to drink enough water. Any ketogenic plan can cause mild or severe dehydration, which could lead to other health complications. Water also helps you lose weight, which is all the more reason to hydrate yourself throughout the day. Have the ingredients ready to make a quick drink on the go. This will help you stay on track and stick to your goals.

Lightning Source UK Ltd.
Milton Keynes UK
UKHW020749110621
385337UK00009B/824